This Log Book Belongs To:

_____

_____

_____

I0420000

Emergency Information:

_____

_____

_____

_____

_____

_____

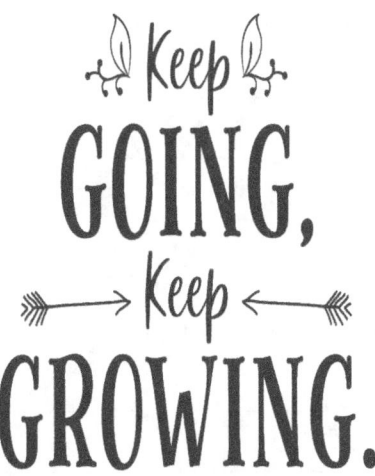

Date: Day:

	Wake	Breakfast	Lunch	Dinner	Bed
Before					
After					
Notes:					

Date: Day:

	Wake	Breakfast	Lunch	Dinner	Bed
Before					
After					
Notes:					

Date: Day:

	Wake	Breakfast	Lunch	Dinner	Bed
Before					
After					
Notes:					

Date: Day:

	Wake	Breakfast	Lunch	Dinner	Bed
Before					
After					
Notes:					

Date: Day:

	Wake	Breakfast	Lunch	Dinner	Bed
Before					
After					
Notes:					

Date: Day:

	Wake	Breakfast	Lunch	Dinner	Bed
Before					
After					
Notes:					

Date: Day:

	Wake	Breakfast	Lunch	Dinner	Bed
Before					
After					
Notes:					

Date: Day:

	Wake	Breakfast	Lunch	Dinner	Bed
Before					
After					
Notes:					

Date: Day:

	Wake	Breakfast	Lunch	Dinner	Bed
Before					
After					
Notes:					

Date: Day:

	Wake	Breakfast	Lunch	Dinner	Bed
Before					
After					
Notes:					

Date: Day:

	Wake	Breakfast	Lunch	Dinner	Bed
Before					
After					
Notes:					

Date: Day:

	Wake	Breakfast	Lunch	Dinner	Bed
Before					
After					
Notes:					

Date: Day:

	Wake	Breakfast	Lunch	Dinner	Bed
Before					
After					
Notes:					

Date: Day:

	Wake	Breakfast	Lunch	Dinner	Bed
Before					
After					
Notes:					

Date: Day:

	Wake	Breakfast	Lunch	Dinner	Bed
Before					
After					
Notes:					

Date: Day:

	Wake	Breakfast	Lunch	Dinner	Bed
Before					
After					
Notes:					

Date: Day:

	Wake	Breakfast	Lunch	Dinner	Bed
Before					
After					
Notes:					

Date: Day:

	Wake	Breakfast	Lunch	Dinner	Bed
Before					
After					
Notes:					

Date: Day:

	Wake	Breakfast	Lunch	Dinner	Bed
Before					
After					
Notes:					

Date: Day:

	Wake	Breakfast	Lunch	Dinner	Bed
Before					
After					
Notes:					

Date: Day:

	Wake	Breakfast	Lunch	Dinner	Bed
Before					
After					
Notes:					

Date: Day:

	Wake	Breakfast	Lunch	Dinner	Bed
Before					
After					
Notes:					

Date: Day:

	Wake	Breakfast	Lunch	Dinner	Bed
Before					
After					
Notes:					

Date: Day:

	Wake	Breakfast	Lunch	Dinner	Bed
Before					
After					
Notes:					

Date: Day:

	Wake	Breakfast	Lunch	Dinner	Bed
Before					
After					
Notes:					

Date: Day:

	Wake	Breakfast	Lunch	Dinner	Bed
Before					
After					
Notes:					

Date: Day:

	Wake	Breakfast	Lunch	Dinner	Bed
Before					
After					
Notes:					

Date: Day:

	Wake	Breakfast	Lunch	Dinner	Bed
Before					
After					
Notes:					

Date: Day:

	Wake	Breakfast	Lunch	Dinner	Bed
Before					
After					
Notes:					

Date: Day:

	Wake	Breakfast	Lunch	Dinner	Bed
Before					
After					
Notes:					

Date: Day:

	Wake	Breakfast	Lunch	Dinner	Bed
Before					
After					
Notes:					

Date: Day:

	Wake	Breakfast	Lunch	Dinner	Bed
Before					
After					
Notes:					

Date: Day:

	Wake	Breakfast	Lunch	Dinner	Bed
Before					
After					
Notes:					

Date: Day:

	Wake	Breakfast	Lunch	Dinner	Bed
Before					
After					
Notes:					

Date: Day:

	Wake	Breakfast	Lunch	Dinner	Bed
Before					
After					
Notes:					

Date: _____ Day: _____

	Wake	Breakfast	Lunch	Dinner	Bed
Before					
After					
Notes:					

Date: _____ Day: _____

	Wake	Breakfast	Lunch	Dinner	Bed
Before					
After					
Notes:					

Date: _____ Day: _____

	Wake	Breakfast	Lunch	Dinner	Bed
Before					
After					
Notes:					

Date: _____ Day: _____

	Wake	Breakfast	Lunch	Dinner	Bed
Before					
After					
Notes:					

Date: _____ Day: _____

	Wake	Breakfast	Lunch	Dinner	Bed
Before					
After					
Notes:					

Date: Day:

	Wake	Breakfast	Lunch	Dinner	Bed
Before					
After					
Notes:					

Date: Day:

	Wake	Breakfast	Lunch	Dinner	Bed
Before					
After					
Notes:					

Date: Day:

	Wake	Breakfast	Lunch	Dinner	Bed
Before					
After					
Notes:					

Date: Day:

	Wake	Breakfast	Lunch	Dinner	Bed
Before					
After					
Notes:					

Date: Day:

	Wake	Breakfast	Lunch	Dinner	Bed
Before					
After					
Notes:					

Date: Day:

	Wake	Breakfast	Lunch	Dinner	Bed
Before					
After					
Notes:					

Date: Day:

	Wake	Breakfast	Lunch	Dinner	Bed
Before					
After					
Notes:					

Date: Day:

	Wake	Breakfast	Lunch	Dinner	Bed
Before					
After					
Notes:					

Date: Day:

	Wake	Breakfast	Lunch	Dinner	Bed
Before					
After					
Notes:					

Date: Day:

	Wake	Breakfast	Lunch	Dinner	Bed
Before					
After					
Notes:					

Date: Day:

	Wake	Breakfast	Lunch	Dinner	Bed
Before					
After					
Notes:					

Date: Day:

	Wake	Breakfast	Lunch	Dinner	Bed
Before					
After					
Notes:					

Date: Day:

	Wake	Breakfast	Lunch	Dinner	Bed
Before					
After					
Notes:					

Date: Day:

	Wake	Breakfast	Lunch	Dinner	Bed
Before					
After					
Notes:					

Date: Day:

	Wake	Breakfast	Lunch	Dinner	Bed
Before					
After					
Notes:					

Date: Day:

	Wake	Breakfast	Lunch	Dinner	Bed
Before					
After					
Notes:					

Date: Day:

	Wake	Breakfast	Lunch	Dinner	Bed
Before					
After					
Notes:					

Date: Day:

	Wake	Breakfast	Lunch	Dinner	Bed
Before					
After					
Notes:					

Date: Day:

	Wake	Breakfast	Lunch	Dinner	Bed
Before					
After					
Notes:					

Date: Day:

	Wake	Breakfast	Lunch	Dinner	Bed
Before					
After					
Notes:					

Date: Day:

	Wake	Breakfast	Lunch	Dinner	Bed
Before					
After					
Notes:					

Date: Day:

	Wake	Breakfast	Lunch	Dinner	Bed
Before					
After					
Notes:					

Date: Day:

	Wake	Breakfast	Lunch	Dinner	Bed
Before					
After					
Notes:					

Date: Day:

	Wake	Breakfast	Lunch	Dinner	Bed
Before					
After					
Notes:					

Date: Day:

	Wake	Breakfast	Lunch	Dinner	Bed
Before					
After					
Notes:					

Date: Day:

	Wake	Breakfast	Lunch	Dinner	Bed
Before					
After					
Notes:					

Date: Day:

	Wake	Breakfast	Lunch	Dinner	Bed
Before					
After					
Notes:					

Date: Day:

	Wake	Breakfast	Lunch	Dinner	Bed
Before					
After					
Notes:					

Date: Day:

	Wake	Breakfast	Lunch	Dinner	Bed
Before					
After					
Notes:					

Date: Day:

	Wake	Breakfast	Lunch	Dinner	Bed
Before					
After					
Notes:					

Date: Day:

	Wake	Breakfast	Lunch	Dinner	Bed
Before					
After					
Notes:					

Date: Day:

	Wake	Breakfast	Lunch	Dinner	Bed
Before					
After					
Notes:					

Date: Day:

	Wake	Breakfast	Lunch	Dinner	Bed
Before					
After					
Notes:					

Date: Day:

	Wake	Breakfast	Lunch	Dinner	Bed
Before					
After					
Notes:					

Date: Day:

	Wake	Breakfast	Lunch	Dinner	Bed
Before					
After					
Notes:					

Date: Day:

	Wake	Breakfast	Lunch	Dinner	Bed
Before					
After					
Notes:					

Date: Day:

	Wake	Breakfast	Lunch	Dinner	Bed
Before					
After					
Notes:					

Date: Day:

	Wake	Breakfast	Lunch	Dinner	Bed
Before					
After					
Notes:					

Date: Day:

	Wake	Breakfast	Lunch	Dinner	Bed
Before					
After					
Notes:					

Date: Day:

	Wake	Breakfast	Lunch	Dinner	Bed
Before					
After					
Notes:					

Date: Day:

	Wake	Breakfast	Lunch	Dinner	Bed
Before					
After					
Notes:					

Date: Day:

	Wake	Breakfast	Lunch	Dinner	Bed
Before					
After					
Notes:					

Date: Day:

	Wake	Breakfast	Lunch	Dinner	Bed
Before					
After					
Notes:					

Date: Day:

	Wake	Breakfast	Lunch	Dinner	Bed
Before					
After					
Notes:					

Date: Day:

	Wake	Breakfast	Lunch	Dinner	Bed
Before					
After					
Notes:					

Date: Day:

	Wake	Breakfast	Lunch	Dinner	Bed
Before					
After					
Notes:					

Date: Day:

	Wake	Breakfast	Lunch	Dinner	Bed
Before					
After					
Notes:					

Date: Day:

	Wake	Breakfast	Lunch	Dinner	Bed
Before					
After					
Notes:					

Date: Day:

	Wake	Breakfast	Lunch	Dinner	Bed
Before					
After					
Notes:					

Date: Day:

	Wake	Breakfast	Lunch	Dinner	Bed
Before					
After					
Notes:					

Date: Day:

	Wake	Breakfast	Lunch	Dinner	Bed
Before					
After					
Notes:					

Date: Day:

	Wake	Breakfast	Lunch	Dinner	Bed
Before					
After					
Notes:					

Date: Day:

	Wake	Breakfast	Lunch	Dinner	Bed
Before					
After					
Notes:					

Date: Day:

	Wake	Breakfast	Lunch	Dinner	Bed
Before					
After					
Notes:					

Date: Day:

	Wake	Breakfast	Lunch	Dinner	Bed
Before					
After					
Notes:					

Date: Day:

	Wake	Breakfast	Lunch	Dinner	Bed
Before					
After					
Notes:					

Date: Day:

	Wake	Breakfast	Lunch	Dinner	Bed
Before					
After					
Notes:					

Date: Day:

	Wake	Breakfast	Lunch	Dinner	Bed
Before					
After					
Notes:					

Date: Day:

	Wake	Breakfast	Lunch	Dinner	Bed
Before					
After					
Notes:					

Date: Day:

	Wake	Breakfast	Lunch	Dinner	Bed
Before					
After					
Notes:					

Date: Day:

	Wake	Breakfast	Lunch	Dinner	Bed
Before					
After					
Notes:					

Date: Day:

	Wake	Breakfast	Lunch	Dinner	Bed
Before					
After					
Notes:					

Date: Day:

	Wake	Breakfast	Lunch	Dinner	Bed
Before					
After					
Notes:					

Date: Day:

	Wake	Breakfast	Lunch	Dinner	Bed
Before					
After					
Notes:					

Date: Day:

	Wake	Breakfast	Lunch	Dinner	Bed
Before					
After					
Notes:					

Date: Day:

	Wake	Breakfast	Lunch	Dinner	Bed
Before					
After					
Notes:					

Date: Day:

	Wake	Breakfast	Lunch	Dinner	Bed
Before					
After					
Notes:					

Date: Day:

	Wake	Breakfast	Lunch	Dinner	Bed
Before					
After					
Notes:					

Date: Day:

	Wake	Breakfast	Lunch	Dinner	Bed
Before					
After					
Notes:					

Date: Day:

	Wake	Breakfast	Lunch	Dinner	Bed
Before					
After					
Notes:					

Date: Day:

	Wake	Breakfast	Lunch	Dinner	Bed
Before					
After					
Notes:					

Date: Day:

	Wake	Breakfast	Lunch	Dinner	Bed
Before					
After					
Notes:					

Date: Day:

	Wake	Breakfast	Lunch	Dinner	Bed
Before					
After					
Notes:					

Date: Day:

	Wake	Breakfast	Lunch	Dinner	Bed
Before					
After					
Notes:					

Date: Day:

	Wake	Breakfast	Lunch	Dinner	Bed
Before					
After					
Notes:					

Date: Day:

	Wake	Breakfast	Lunch	Dinner	Bed
Before					
After					
Notes:					

Date: Day:

	Wake	Breakfast	Lunch	Dinner	Bed
Before					
After					
Notes:					

Date: Day:

	Wake	Breakfast	Lunch	Dinner	Bed
Before					
After					
Notes:					

Date: Day:

	Wake	Breakfast	Lunch	Dinner	Bed
Before					
After					
Notes:					

Date: Day:

	Wake	Breakfast	Lunch	Dinner	Bed
Before					
After					
Notes:					

Date: Day:

	Wake	Breakfast	Lunch	Dinner	Bed
Before					
After					
Notes:					

Date: Day:

	Wake	Breakfast	Lunch	Dinner	Bed
Before					
After					
Notes:					

Date: Day:

	Wake	Breakfast	Lunch	Dinner	Bed
Before					
After					
Notes:					

Date: Day:

	Wake	Breakfast	Lunch	Dinner	Bed
Before					
After					
Notes:					

Date: Day:

	Wake	Breakfast	Lunch	Dinner	Bed
Before					
After					
Notes:					

Date: Day:

	Wake	Breakfast	Lunch	Dinner	Bed
Before					
After					
Notes:					

Date: Day:

	Wake	Breakfast	Lunch	Dinner	Bed
Before					
After					
Notes:					

Date: Day:

	Wake	Breakfast	Lunch	Dinner	Bed
Before					
After					
Notes:					

Date: Day:

	Wake	Breakfast	Lunch	Dinner	Bed
Before					
After					
Notes:					

Date: Day:

	Wake	Breakfast	Lunch	Dinner	Bed
Before					
After					
Notes:					

Date: Day:

	Wake	Breakfast	Lunch	Dinner	Bed
Before					
After					
Notes:					

Date: Day:

	Wake	Breakfast	Lunch	Dinner	Bed
Before					
After					
Notes:					

Date: Day:

	Wake	Breakfast	Lunch	Dinner	Bed
Before					
After					
Notes:					

Date: Day:

	Wake	Breakfast	Lunch	Dinner	Bed
Before					
After					
Notes:					

Date: Day:

	Wake	Breakfast	Lunch	Dinner	Bed
Before					
After					
Notes:					

Date: Day:

	Wake	Breakfast	Lunch	Dinner	Bed
Before					
After					
Notes:					

Date: Day:

	Wake	Breakfast	Lunch	Dinner	Bed
Before					
After					
Notes:					

Date: Day:

	Wake	Breakfast	Lunch	Dinner	Bed
Before					
After					
Notes:					

Date: Day:

	Wake	Breakfast	Lunch	Dinner	Bed
Before					
After					
Notes:					

Date: Day:

	Wake	Breakfast	Lunch	Dinner	Bed
Before					
After					
Notes:					

Date: Day:

	Wake	Breakfast	Lunch	Dinner	Bed
Before					
After					
Notes:					

Date: Day:

	Wake	Breakfast	Lunch	Dinner	Bed
Before					
After					
Notes:					

Date: Day:

	Wake	Breakfast	Lunch	Dinner	Bed
Before					
After					
Notes:					

Date: Day:

	Wake	Breakfast	Lunch	Dinner	Bed
Before					
After					
Notes:					

Date: Day:

	Wake	Breakfast	Lunch	Dinner	Bed
Before					
After					
Notes:					

Date: Day:

	Wake	Breakfast	Lunch	Dinner	Bed
Before					
After					
Notes:					

Date: Day:

	Wake	Breakfast	Lunch	Dinner	Bed
Before					
After					
Notes:					

Date: Day:

	Wake	Breakfast	Lunch	Dinner	Bed
Before					
After					
Notes:					

Date: Day:

	Wake	Breakfast	Lunch	Dinner	Bed
Before					
After					
Notes:					

Date: Day:

	Wake	Breakfast	Lunch	Dinner	Bed
Before					
After					
Notes:					

Date: Day:

	Wake	Breakfast	Lunch	Dinner	Bed
Before					
After					
Notes:					

Date: Day:

	Wake	Breakfast	Lunch	Dinner	Bed
Before					
After					
Notes:					

Date: Day:

	Wake	Breakfast	Lunch	Dinner	Bed
Before					
After					
Notes:					

Date: Day:

	Wake	Breakfast	Lunch	Dinner	Bed
Before					
After					
Notes:					

Date: Day:

	Wake	Breakfast	Lunch	Dinner	Bed
Before					
After					
Notes:					

Date: Day:

	Wake	Breakfast	Lunch	Dinner	Bed
Before					
After					
Notes:					

Date: Day:

	Wake	Breakfast	Lunch	Dinner	Bed
Before					
After					
Notes:					

Date: Day:

	Wake	Breakfast	Lunch	Dinner	Bed
Before					
After					
Notes:					

Date: Day:

	Wake	Breakfast	Lunch	Dinner	Bed
Before					
After					
Notes:					

Date: Day:

	Wake	Breakfast	Lunch	Dinner	Bed
Before					
After					
Notes:					

Date: Day:

	Wake	Breakfast	Lunch	Dinner	Bed
Before					
After					
Notes:					

Date: Day:

	Wake	Breakfast	Lunch	Dinner	Bed
Before					
After					
Notes:					

Date: Day:

	Wake	Breakfast	Lunch	Dinner	Bed
Before					
After					
Notes:					

Date: Day:

	Wake	Breakfast	Lunch	Dinner	Bed
Before					
After					
Notes:					

Date: Day:

	Wake	Breakfast	Lunch	Dinner	Bed
Before					
After					
Notes:					

Date: Day:

	Wake	Breakfast	Lunch	Dinner	Bed
Before					
After					
Notes:					

Date: Day:

	Wake	Breakfast	Lunch	Dinner	Bed
Before					
After					
Notes:					

Date: Day:

	Wake	Breakfast	Lunch	Dinner	Bed
Before					
After					
Notes:					

Date: Day:

	Wake	Breakfast	Lunch	Dinner	Bed
Before					
After					
Notes:					

Date: Day:

	Wake	Breakfast	Lunch	Dinner	Bed
Before					
After					
Notes:					

Date: Day:

	Wake	Breakfast	Lunch	Dinner	Bed
Before					
After					
Notes:					

Date: Day:

	Wake	Breakfast	Lunch	Dinner	Bed
Before					
After					
Notes:					

Date: Day:

	Wake	Breakfast	Lunch	Dinner	Bed
Before					
After					
Notes:					

Date: Day:

	Wake	Breakfast	Lunch	Dinner	Bed
Before					
After					
Notes:					

Date: Day:

	Wake	Breakfast	Lunch	Dinner	Bed
Before					
After					
Notes:					

Date: Day:

	Wake	Breakfast	Lunch	Dinner	Bed
Before					
After					
Notes:					

Date: Day:

	Wake	Breakfast	Lunch	Dinner	Bed
Before					
After					
Notes:					

Date: Day:

	Wake	Breakfast	Lunch	Dinner	Bed
Before					
After					
Notes:					

Date: Day:

	Wake	Breakfast	Lunch	Dinner	Bed
Before					
After					
Notes:					

Date: Day:

	Wake	Breakfast	Lunch	Dinner	Bed
Before					
After					
Notes:					

Date: Day:

	Wake	Breakfast	Lunch	Dinner	Bed
Before					
After					
Notes:					

Date: Day:

	Wake	Breakfast	Lunch	Dinner	Bed
Before					
After					
Notes:					

Date: Day:

	Wake	Breakfast	Lunch	Dinner	Bed
Before					
After					
Notes:					

Date: Day:

	Wake	Breakfast	Lunch	Dinner	Bed
Before					
After					
Notes:					

Date: Day:

	Wake	Breakfast	Lunch	Dinner	Bed
Before					
After					
Notes:					

Date: Day:

	Wake	Breakfast	Lunch	Dinner	Bed
Before					
After					
Notes:					

Date: Day:

	Wake	Breakfast	Lunch	Dinner	Bed
Before					
After					
Notes:					

Date: Day:

	Wake	Breakfast	Lunch	Dinner	Bed
Before					
After					
Notes:					

Date: Day:

	Wake	Breakfast	Lunch	Dinner	Bed
Before					
After					
Notes:					

Date: Day:

	Wake	Breakfast	Lunch	Dinner	Bed
Before					
After					
Notes:					

Date: _____ Day: _____

	Wake	Breakfast	Lunch	Dinner	Bed
Before					
After					
Notes:					

Date: _____ Day: _____

	Wake	Breakfast	Lunch	Dinner	Bed
Before					
After					
Notes:					

Date: _____ Day: _____

	Wake	Breakfast	Lunch	Dinner	Bed
Before					
After					
Notes:					

Date: _____ Day: _____

	Wake	Breakfast	Lunch	Dinner	Bed
Before					
After					
Notes:					

Date: _____ Day: _____

	Wake	Breakfast	Lunch	Dinner	Bed
Before					
After					
Notes:					

Date: Day:

	Wake	Breakfast	Lunch	Dinner	Bed
Before					
After					
Notes:					

Date: Day:

	Wake	Breakfast	Lunch	Dinner	Bed
Before					
After					
Notes:					

Date: Day:

	Wake	Breakfast	Lunch	Dinner	Bed
Before					
After					
Notes:					

Date: Day:

	Wake	Breakfast	Lunch	Dinner	Bed
Before					
After					
Notes:					

Date: Day:

	Wake	Breakfast	Lunch	Dinner	Bed
Before					
After					
Notes:					

Date: Day:

	Wake	Breakfast	Lunch	Dinner	Bed
Before					
After					
Notes:					

Date: Day:

	Wake	Breakfast	Lunch	Dinner	Bed
Before					
After					
Notes:					

Date: Day:

	Wake	Breakfast	Lunch	Dinner	Bed
Before					
After					
Notes:					

Date: Day:

	Wake	Breakfast	Lunch	Dinner	Bed
Before					
After					
Notes:					

Date: Day:

	Wake	Breakfast	Lunch	Dinner	Bed
Before					
After					
Notes:					

Date: Day:

	Wake	Breakfast	Lunch	Dinner	Bed
Before					
After					
Notes:					

Date: Day:

	Wake	Breakfast	Lunch	Dinner	Bed
Before					
After					
Notes:					

Date: Day:

	Wake	Breakfast	Lunch	Dinner	Bed
Before					
After					
Notes:					

Date: Day:

	Wake	Breakfast	Lunch	Dinner	Bed
Before					
After					
Notes:					

Date: Day:

	Wake	Breakfast	Lunch	Dinner	Bed
Before					
After					
Notes:					

Date: Day:

	Wake	Breakfast	Lunch	Dinner	Bed
Before					
After					
Notes:					

Date: Day:

	Wake	Breakfast	Lunch	Dinner	Bed
Before					
After					
Notes:					

Date: Day:

	Wake	Breakfast	Lunch	Dinner	Bed
Before					
After					
Notes:					

Date: Day:

	Wake	Breakfast	Lunch	Dinner	Bed
Before					
After					
Notes:					

Date: Day:

	Wake	Breakfast	Lunch	Dinner	Bed
Before					
After					
Notes:					

Date: Day:

	Wake	Breakfast	Lunch	Dinner	Bed
Before					
After					
Notes:					

Date: Day:

	Wake	Breakfast	Lunch	Dinner	Bed
Before					
After					
Notes:					

Date: Day:

	Wake	Breakfast	Lunch	Dinner	Bed
Before					
After					
Notes:					

Date: Day:

	Wake	Breakfast	Lunch	Dinner	Bed
Before					
After					
Notes:					

Date: Day:

	Wake	Breakfast	Lunch	Dinner	Bed
Before					
After					
Notes:					

Date: Day:

	Wake	Breakfast	Lunch	Dinner	Bed
Before					
After					
Notes:					

Date: Day:

	Wake	Breakfast	Lunch	Dinner	Bed
Before					
After					
Notes:					

Date: Day:

	Wake	Breakfast	Lunch	Dinner	Bed
Before					
After					
Notes:					

Date: Day:

	Wake	Breakfast	Lunch	Dinner	Bed
Before					
After					
Notes:					

Date: Day:

	Wake	Breakfast	Lunch	Dinner	Bed
Before					
After					
Notes:					

Date: Day:

	Wake	Breakfast	Lunch	Dinner	Bed
Before					
After					
Notes:					

Date: Day:

	Wake	Breakfast	Lunch	Dinner	Bed
Before					
After					
Notes:					

Date: Day:

	Wake	Breakfast	Lunch	Dinner	Bed
Before					
After					
Notes:					

Date: Day:

	Wake	Breakfast	Lunch	Dinner	Bed
Before					
After					
Notes:					

Date: Day:

	Wake	Breakfast	Lunch	Dinner	Bed
Before					
After					
Notes:					

Date: Day:

	Wake	Breakfast	Lunch	Dinner	Bed
Before					
After					
Notes:					

Date: Day:

	Wake	Breakfast	Lunch	Dinner	Bed
Before					
After					
Notes:					

Date: Day:

	Wake	Breakfast	Lunch	Dinner	Bed
Before					
After					
Notes:					

Date: Day:

	Wake	Breakfast	Lunch	Dinner	Bed
Before					
After					
Notes:					

Date: Day:

	Wake	Breakfast	Lunch	Dinner	Bed
Before					
After					
Notes:					

Date: Day:

	Wake	Breakfast	Lunch	Dinner	Bed
Before					
After					
Notes:					

Date: Day:

	Wake	Breakfast	Lunch	Dinner	Bed
Before					
After					
Notes:					

Date: Day:

	Wake	Breakfast	Lunch	Dinner	Bed
Before					
After					
Notes:					

Date: Day:

	Wake	Breakfast	Lunch	Dinner	Bed
Before					
After					
Notes:					

Date: Day:

	Wake	Breakfast	Lunch	Dinner	Bed
Before					
After					
Notes:					

Date: Day:

	Wake	Breakfast	Lunch	Dinner	Bed
Before					
After					
Notes:					

Date: Day:

	Wake	Breakfast	Lunch	Dinner	Bed
Before					
After					
Notes:					

Date: Day:

	Wake	Breakfast	Lunch	Dinner	Bed
Before					
After					
Notes:					

Date: Day:

	Wake	Breakfast	Lunch	Dinner	Bed
Before					
After					
Notes:					

Date: Day:

	Wake	Breakfast	Lunch	Dinner	Bed
Before					
After					
Notes:					

Date: Day:

	Wake	Breakfast	Lunch	Dinner	Bed
Before					
After					
Notes:					

Date: Day:

	Wake	Breakfast	Lunch	Dinner	Bed
Before					
After					
Notes:					

Date: Day:

	Wake	Breakfast	Lunch	Dinner	Bed
Before					
After					
Notes:					

Date: Day:

	Wake	Breakfast	Lunch	Dinner	Bed
Before					
After					
Notes:					

Date: Day:

	Wake	Breakfast	Lunch	Dinner	Bed
Before					
After					
Notes:					

Date: Day:

	Wake	Breakfast	Lunch	Dinner	Bed
Before					
After					
Notes:					

Date: Day:

	Wake	Breakfast	Lunch	Dinner	Bed
Before					
After					
Notes:					

Date: Day:

	Wake	Breakfast	Lunch	Dinner	Bed
Before					
After					
Notes:					

Date: Day:

	Wake	Breakfast	Lunch	Dinner	Bed
Before					
After					
Notes:					

Date: Day:

	Wake	Breakfast	Lunch	Dinner	Bed
Before					
After					
Notes:					

Date: Day:

	Wake	Breakfast	Lunch	Dinner	Bed
Before					
After					
Notes:					

Date: Day:

	Wake	Breakfast	Lunch	Dinner	Bed
Before					
After					
Notes:					

Date: Day:

	Wake	Breakfast	Lunch	Dinner	Bed
Before					
After					
Notes:					

Date: Day:

	Wake	Breakfast	Lunch	Dinner	Bed
Before					
After					
Notes:					

Date: Day:

	Wake	Breakfast	Lunch	Dinner	Bed
Before					
After					
Notes:					

Date: Day:

	Wake	Breakfast	Lunch	Dinner	Bed
Before					
After					
Notes:					

Date: Day:

	Wake	Breakfast	Lunch	Dinner	Bed
Before					
After					
Notes:					

Date: Day:

	Wake	Breakfast	Lunch	Dinner	Bed
Before					
After					
Notes:					

Date: Day:

	Wake	Breakfast	Lunch	Dinner	Bed
Before					
After					
Notes:					

Date: Day:

	Wake	Breakfast	Lunch	Dinner	Bed
Before					
After					
Notes:					

Date: Day:

	Wake	Breakfast	Lunch	Dinner	Bed
Before					
After					
Notes:					

Date: Day:

	Wake	Breakfast	Lunch	Dinner	Bed
Before					
After					
Notes:					

Date: Day:

	Wake	Breakfast	Lunch	Dinner	Bed
Before					
After					
Notes:					

Date: Day:

	Wake	Breakfast	Lunch	Dinner	Bed
Before					
After					
Notes:					

Date: Day:

	Wake	Breakfast	Lunch	Dinner	Bed
Before					
After					
Notes:					

Date: Day:

	Wake	Breakfast	Lunch	Dinner	Bed
Before					
After					
Notes:					

Date: Day:

	Wake	Breakfast	Lunch	Dinner	Bed
Before					
After					
Notes:					

Date: Day:

	Wake	Breakfast	Lunch	Dinner	Bed
Before					
After					
Notes:					

Date: Day:

	Wake	Breakfast	Lunch	Dinner	Bed
Before					
After					
Notes:					

Date: Day:

	Wake	Breakfast	Lunch	Dinner	Bed
Before					
After					
Notes:					

Date: Day:

	Wake	Breakfast	Lunch	Dinner	Bed
Before					
After					
Notes:					

Date: Day:

	Wake	Breakfast	Lunch	Dinner	Bed
Before					
After					
Notes:					

Date: Day:

	Wake	Breakfast	Lunch	Dinner	Bed
Before					
After					
Notes:					

Date: Day:

	Wake	Breakfast	Lunch	Dinner	Bed
Before					
After					
Notes:					

Date: Day:

	Wake	Breakfast	Lunch	Dinner	Bed
Before					
After					
Notes:					

Date: Day:

	Wake	Breakfast	Lunch	Dinner	Bed
Before					
After					
Notes:					

Date: Day:

	Wake	Breakfast	Lunch	Dinner	Bed
Before					
After					
Notes:					

Date: Day:

	Wake	Breakfast	Lunch	Dinner	Bed
Before					
After					
Notes:					

Date: Day:

	Wake	Breakfast	Lunch	Dinner	Bed
Before					
After					
Notes:					

Date: Day:

	Wake	Breakfast	Lunch	Dinner	Bed
Before					
After					
Notes:					

Date: Day:

	Wake	Breakfast	Lunch	Dinner	Bed
Before					
After					
Notes:					

Date: Day:

	Wake	Breakfast	Lunch	Dinner	Bed
Before					
After					
Notes:					

Date: Day:

	Wake	Breakfast	Lunch	Dinner	Bed
Before					
After					
Notes:					

Date: Day:

	Wake	Breakfast	Lunch	Dinner	Bed
Before					
After					
Notes:					

Date: Day:

	Wake	Breakfast	Lunch	Dinner	Bed
Before					
After					
Notes:					

Date: Day:

	Wake	Breakfast	Lunch	Dinner	Bed
Before					
After					
Notes:					

Date: Day:

	Wake	Breakfast	Lunch	Dinner	Bed
Before					
After					
Notes:					

Date: Day:

	Wake	Breakfast	Lunch	Dinner	Bed
Before					
After					
Notes:					

Date: Day:

	Wake	Breakfast	Lunch	Dinner	Bed
Before					
After					
Notes:					

Date: Day:

	Wake	Breakfast	Lunch	Dinner	Bed
Before					
After					
Notes:					

Date: Day:

	Wake	Breakfast	Lunch	Dinner	Bed
Before					
After					
Notes:					

Date: Day:

	Wake	Breakfast	Lunch	Dinner	Bed
Before					
After					
Notes:					

Date: Day:

	Wake	Breakfast	Lunch	Dinner	Bed
Before					
After					
Notes:					

Date: Day:

	Wake	Breakfast	Lunch	Dinner	Bed
Before					
After					
Notes:					

Date: Day:

	Wake	Breakfast	Lunch	Dinner	Bed
Before					
After					
Notes:					

Date: Day:

	Wake	Breakfast	Lunch	Dinner	Bed
Before					
After					
Notes:					

Date: Day:

	Wake	Breakfast	Lunch	Dinner	Bed
Before					
After					
Notes:					

Date: Day:

	Wake	Breakfast	Lunch	Dinner	Bed
Before					
After					
Notes:					

Date: Day:

	Wake	Breakfast	Lunch	Dinner	Bed
Before					
After					
Notes:					

Date: Day:

	Wake	Breakfast	Lunch	Dinner	Bed
Before					
After					
Notes:					

Date: Day:

	Wake	Breakfast	Lunch	Dinner	Bed
Before					
After					
Notes:					

Date: Day:

	Wake	Breakfast	Lunch	Dinner	Bed
Before					
After					
Notes:					

Date: Day:

	Wake	Breakfast	Lunch	Dinner	Bed
Before					
After					
Notes:					

Date: Day:

	Wake	Breakfast	Lunch	Dinner	Bed
Before					
After					
Notes:					

Date: Day:

	Wake	Breakfast	Lunch	Dinner	Bed
Before					
After					
Notes:					

Date: Day:

	Wake	Breakfast	Lunch	Dinner	Bed
Before					
After					
Notes:					

Date: Day:

	Wake	Breakfast	Lunch	Dinner	Bed
Before					
After					
Notes:					

Date: Day:

	Wake	Breakfast	Lunch	Dinner	Bed
Before					
After					
Notes:					

Date: Day:

	Wake	Breakfast	Lunch	Dinner	Bed
Before					
After					
Notes:					

Date: Day:

	Wake	Breakfast	Lunch	Dinner	Bed
Before					
After					
Notes:					

Date: Day:

	Wake	Breakfast	Lunch	Dinner	Bed
Before					
After					
Notes:					

Date: Day:

	Wake	Breakfast	Lunch	Dinner	Bed
Before					
After					
Notes:					

Date: Day:

	Wake	Breakfast	Lunch	Dinner	Bed
Before					
After					
Notes:					

Date: Day:

	Wake	Breakfast	Lunch	Dinner	Bed
Before					
After					
Notes:					

Date: Day:

	Wake	Breakfast	Lunch	Dinner	Bed
Before					
After					
Notes:					

Date: Day:

	Wake	Breakfast	Lunch	Dinner	Bed
Before					
After					
Notes:					

Date: Day:

	Wake	Breakfast	Lunch	Dinner	Bed
Before					
After					
Notes:					

Date: Day:

	Wake	Breakfast	Lunch	Dinner	Bed
Before					
After					
Notes:					

Date: Day:

	Wake	Breakfast	Lunch	Dinner	Bed
Before					
After					
Notes:					

Date: Day:

	Wake	Breakfast	Lunch	Dinner	Bed
Before					
After					
Notes:					

Date: Day:

	Wake	Breakfast	Lunch	Dinner	Bed
Before					
After					
Notes:					

Date: Day:

	Wake	Breakfast	Lunch	Dinner	Bed
Before					
After					
Notes:					

Date: Day:

	Wake	Breakfast	Lunch	Dinner	Bed
Before					
After					
Notes:					

Date: Day:

	Wake	Breakfast	Lunch	Dinner	Bed
Before					
After					
Notes:					

Date: Day:

	Wake	Breakfast	Lunch	Dinner	Bed
Before					
After					
Notes:					

Date: Day:

	Wake	Breakfast	Lunch	Dinner	Bed
Before					
After					
Notes:					

Date: Day:

	Wake	Breakfast	Lunch	Dinner	Bed
Before					
After					
Notes:					

Date: Day:

	Wake	Breakfast	Lunch	Dinner	Bed
Before					
After					
Notes:					

Date: Day:

	Wake	Breakfast	Lunch	Dinner	Bed
Before					
After					
Notes:					

Date: Day:

	Wake	Breakfast	Lunch	Dinner	Bed
Before					
After					
Notes:					

Date: Day:

	Wake	Breakfast	Lunch	Dinner	Bed
Before					
After					
Notes:					

Date: Day:

	Wake	Breakfast	Lunch	Dinner	Bed
Before					
After					
Notes:					

Date: Day:

	Wake	Breakfast	Lunch	Dinner	Bed
Before					
After					
Notes:					

Date: Day:

	Wake	Breakfast	Lunch	Dinner	Bed
Before					
After					
Notes:					

Date: Day:

	Wake	Breakfast	Lunch	Dinner	Bed
Before					
After					
Notes:					

Date: Day:

	Wake	Breakfast	Lunch	Dinner	Bed
Before					
After					
Notes:					

Date: Day:

	Wake	Breakfast	Lunch	Dinner	Bed
Before					
After					
Notes:					

Date: Day:

	Wake	Breakfast	Lunch	Dinner	Bed
Before					
After					
Notes:					

Date: Day:

	Wake	Breakfast	Lunch	Dinner	Bed
Before					
After					
Notes:					

Date: Day:

	Wake	Breakfast	Lunch	Dinner	Bed
Before					
After					
Notes:					

Date: Day:

	Wake	Breakfast	Lunch	Dinner	Bed
Before					
After					
Notes:					

Date: Day:

	Wake	Breakfast	Lunch	Dinner	Bed
Before					
After					
Notes:					

Date: Day:

	Wake	Breakfast	Lunch	Dinner	Bed
Before					
After					
Notes:					

Date: Day:

	Wake	Breakfast	Lunch	Dinner	Bed
Before					
After					
Notes:					

Date: Day:

	Wake	Breakfast	Lunch	Dinner	Bed
Before					
After					
Notes:					

Date: Day:

	Wake	Breakfast	Lunch	Dinner	Bed
Before					
After					
Notes:					

Date: Day:

	Wake	Breakfast	Lunch	Dinner	Bed
Before					
After					
Notes:					

Date: Day:

	Wake	Breakfast	Lunch	Dinner	Bed
Before					
After					
Notes:					

Date: Day:

	Wake	Breakfast	Lunch	Dinner	Bed
Before					
After					
Notes:					

Date: Day:

	Wake	Breakfast	Lunch	Dinner	Bed
Before					
After					
Notes:					

Date: Day:

	Wake	Breakfast	Lunch	Dinner	Bed
Before					
After					
Notes:					

Date: Day:

	Wake	Breakfast	Lunch	Dinner	Bed
Before					
After					
Notes:					

Date: Day:

	Wake	Breakfast	Lunch	Dinner	Bed
Before					
After					
Notes:					

Date: Day:

	Wake	Breakfast	Lunch	Dinner	Bed
Before					
After					
Notes:					

Date: Day:

	Wake	Breakfast	Lunch	Dinner	Bed
Before					
After					
Notes:					

Date: Day:

	Wake	Breakfast	Lunch	Dinner	Bed
Before					
After					
Notes:					

Date: Day:

	Wake	Breakfast	Lunch	Dinner	Bed
Before					
After					
Notes:					

Date: Day:

	Wake	Breakfast	Lunch	Dinner	Bed
Before					
After					
Notes:					

Date: Day:

	Wake	Breakfast	Lunch	Dinner	Bed
Before					
After					
Notes:					

Date: Day:

	Wake	Breakfast	Lunch	Dinner	Bed
Before					
After					
Notes:					

Date: Day:

	Wake	Breakfast	Lunch	Dinner	Bed
Before					
After					
Notes:					

Date: Day:

	Wake	Breakfast	Lunch	Dinner	Bed
Before					
After					
Notes:					

Date: Day:

	Wake	Breakfast	Lunch	Dinner	Bed
Before					
After					
Notes:					

Date: Day:

	Wake	Breakfast	Lunch	Dinner	Bed
Before					
After					
Notes:					

Date: Day:

	Wake	Breakfast	Lunch	Dinner	Bed
Before					
After					
Notes:					

Date: Day:

	Wake	Breakfast	Lunch	Dinner	Bed
Before					
After					
Notes:					

Date: Day:

	Wake	Breakfast	Lunch	Dinner	Bed
Before					
After					
Notes:					

Date: Day:

	Wake	Breakfast	Lunch	Dinner	Bed
Before					
After					
Notes:					

Date: Day:

	Wake	Breakfast	Lunch	Dinner	Bed
Before					
After					
Notes:					

Date: Day:

	Wake	Breakfast	Lunch	Dinner	Bed
Before					
After					
Notes:					

Date: Day:

	Wake	Breakfast	Lunch	Dinner	Bed
Before					
After					
Notes:					

Date: Day:

	Wake	Breakfast	Lunch	Dinner	Bed
Before					
After					
Notes:					

Date: Day:

	Wake	Breakfast	Lunch	Dinner	Bed
Before					
After					
Notes:					

Date: Day:

	Wake	Breakfast	Lunch	Dinner	Bed
Before					
After					
Notes:					

Date: Day:

	Wake	Breakfast	Lunch	Dinner	Bed
Before					
After					
Notes:					

Date: Day:

	Wake	Breakfast	Lunch	Dinner	Bed
Before					
After					
Notes:					

Date: Day:

	Wake	Breakfast	Lunch	Dinner	Bed
Before					
After					
Notes:					

Date: Day:

	Wake	Breakfast	Lunch	Dinner	Bed
Before					
After					
Notes:					

Date: Day:

	Wake	Breakfast	Lunch	Dinner	Bed
Before					
After					
Notes:					

Date: Day:

	Wake	Breakfast	Lunch	Dinner	Bed
Before					
After					
Notes:					

Date: Day:

	Wake	Breakfast	Lunch	Dinner	Bed
Before					
After					
Notes:					

Date: Day:

	Wake	Breakfast	Lunch	Dinner	Bed
Before					
After					
Notes:					

Date: Day:

	Wake	Breakfast	Lunch	Dinner	Bed
Before					
After					
Notes:					

Date: Day:

	Wake	Breakfast	Lunch	Dinner	Bed
Before					
After					
Notes:					

Date: Day:

	Wake	Breakfast	Lunch	Dinner	Bed
Before					
After					
Notes:					

Date: Day:

	Wake	Breakfast	Lunch	Dinner	Bed
Before					
After					
Notes:					

Date: Day:

	Wake	Breakfast	Lunch	Dinner	Bed
Before					
After					
Notes:					

Date: Day:

	Wake	Breakfast	Lunch	Dinner	Bed
Before					
After					
Notes:					

Date: Day:

	Wake	Breakfast	Lunch	Dinner	Bed
Before					
After					
Notes:					

Date: Day:

	Wake	Breakfast	Lunch	Dinner	Bed
Before					
After					
Notes:					

Date: Day:

	Wake	Breakfast	Lunch	Dinner	Bed
Before					
After					
Notes:					

Date: Day:

	Wake	Breakfast	Lunch	Dinner	Bed
Before					
After					
Notes:					

Date: Day:

	Wake	Breakfast	Lunch	Dinner	Bed
Before					
After					
Notes:					

Date: Day:

	Wake	Breakfast	Lunch	Dinner	Bed
Before					
After					
Notes:					

Date: Day:

	Wake	Breakfast	Lunch	Dinner	Bed
Before					
After					
Notes:					

Date: Day:

	Wake	Breakfast	Lunch	Dinner	Bed
Before					
After					
Notes:					

Date: Day:

	Wake	Breakfast	Lunch	Dinner	Bed
Before					
After					
Notes:					

Date: Day:

	Wake	Breakfast	Lunch	Dinner	Bed
Before					
After					
Notes:					

Date: Day:

	Wake	Breakfast	Lunch	Dinner	Bed
Before					
After					
Notes:					

Date: Day:

	Wake	Breakfast	Lunch	Dinner	Bed
Before					
After					
Notes:					

Date: Day:

	Wake	Breakfast	Lunch	Dinner	Bed
Before					
After					
Notes:					

Date: Day:

	Wake	Breakfast	Lunch	Dinner	Bed
Before					
After					
Notes:					

Date: Day:

	Wake	Breakfast	Lunch	Dinner	Bed
Before					
After					
Notes:					

Date: Day:

	Wake	Breakfast	Lunch	Dinner	Bed
Before					
After					
Notes:					

Date: Day:

	Wake	Breakfast	Lunch	Dinner	Bed
Before					
After					
Notes:					

Date: Day:

	Wake	Breakfast	Lunch	Dinner	Bed
Before					
After					
Notes:					

Date: Day:

	Wake	Breakfast	Lunch	Dinner	Bed
Before					
After					
Notes:					

Date: Day:

	Wake	Breakfast	Lunch	Dinner	Bed
Before					
After					
Notes:					

Date: Day:

	Wake	Breakfast	Lunch	Dinner	Bed
Before					
After					
Notes:					

Date: Day:

	Wake	Breakfast	Lunch	Dinner	Bed
Before					
After					
Notes:					

Date: Day:

	Wake	Breakfast	Lunch	Dinner	Bed
Before					
After					
Notes:					

Date: Day:

	Wake	Breakfast	Lunch	Dinner	Bed
Before					
After					
Notes:					

Date: Day:

	Wake	Breakfast	Lunch	Dinner	Bed
Before					
After					
Notes:					

Date: Day:

	Wake	Breakfast	Lunch	Dinner	Bed
Before					
After					
Notes:					

Date: Day:

	Wake	Breakfast	Lunch	Dinner	Bed
Before					
After					
Notes:					

Date: Day:

	Wake	Breakfast	Lunch	Dinner	Bed
Before					
After					
Notes:					

Date: Day:

	Wake	Breakfast	Lunch	Dinner	Bed
Before					
After					
Notes:					

Date: Day:

	Wake	Breakfast	Lunch	Dinner	Bed
Before					
After					
Notes:					

Date: Day:

	Wake	Breakfast	Lunch	Dinner	Bed
Before					
After					
Notes:					

Date: Day:

	Wake	Breakfast	Lunch	Dinner	Bed
Before					
After					
Notes:					

Date: Day:

	Wake	Breakfast	Lunch	Dinner	Bed
Before					
After					
Notes:					

Date: Day:

	Wake	Breakfast	Lunch	Dinner	Bed
Before					
After					
Notes:					

Date: Day:

	Wake	Breakfast	Lunch	Dinner	Bed
Before					
After					
Notes:					

Date: Day:

	Wake	Breakfast	Lunch	Dinner	Bed
Before					
After					
Notes:					

Date: Day:

	Wake	Breakfast	Lunch	Dinner	Bed
Before					
After					
Notes:					

Date: Day:

	Wake	Breakfast	Lunch	Dinner	Bed
Before					
After					
Notes:					

Date: Day:

	Wake	Breakfast	Lunch	Dinner	Bed
Before					
After					
Notes:					

Date: Day:

	Wake	Breakfast	Lunch	Dinner	Bed
Before					
After					
Notes:					

Date: Day:

	Wake	Breakfast	Lunch	Dinner	Bed
Before					
After					
Notes:					

Date: Day:

	Wake	Breakfast	Lunch	Dinner	Bed
Before					
After					
Notes:					

Date: Day:

	Wake	Breakfast	Lunch	Dinner	Bed
Before					
After					
Notes:					

Date: Day:

	Wake	Breakfast	Lunch	Dinner	Bed
Before					
After					
Notes:					

Date: Day:

	Wake	Breakfast	Lunch	Dinner	Bed
Before					
After					
Notes:					

Date: Day:

	Wake	Breakfast	Lunch	Dinner	Bed
Before					
After					
Notes:					

Date: Day:

	Wake	Breakfast	Lunch	Dinner	Bed
Before					
After					
Notes:					

Date: _____ Day: _____

	Wake	Breakfast	Lunch	Dinner	Bed
Before					
After					
Notes:					

Date: _____ Day: _____

	Wake	Breakfast	Lunch	Dinner	Bed
Before					
After					
Notes:					

Date: _____ Day: _____

	Wake	Breakfast	Lunch	Dinner	Bed
Before					
After					
Notes:					

Date: _____ Day: _____

	Wake	Breakfast	Lunch	Dinner	Bed
Before					
After					
Notes:					

Date: _____ Day: _____

	Wake	Breakfast	Lunch	Dinner	Bed
Before					
After					
Notes:					

Date: Day:

	Wake	Breakfast	Lunch	Dinner	Bed
Before					
After					
Notes:					

Date: Day:

	Wake	Breakfast	Lunch	Dinner	Bed
Before					
After					
Notes:					

Date: Day:

	Wake	Breakfast	Lunch	Dinner	Bed
Before					
After					
Notes:					

Date: Day:

	Wake	Breakfast	Lunch	Dinner	Bed
Before					
After					
Notes:					

Date: Day:

	Wake	Breakfast	Lunch	Dinner	Bed
Before					
After					
Notes:					

Date: Day:

	Wake	Breakfast	Lunch	Dinner	Bed
Before					
After					
Notes:					

Date: Day:

	Wake	Breakfast	Lunch	Dinner	Bed
Before					
After					
Notes:					

Date: Day:

	Wake	Breakfast	Lunch	Dinner	Bed
Before					
After					
Notes:					

Date: Day:

	Wake	Breakfast	Lunch	Dinner	Bed
Before					
After					
Notes:					

Date: Day:

	Wake	Breakfast	Lunch	Dinner	Bed
Before					
After					
Notes:					

Date: Day:

	Wake	Breakfast	Lunch	Dinner	Bed
Before					
After					
Notes:					

Date: Day:

	Wake	Breakfast	Lunch	Dinner	Bed
Before					
After					
Notes:					

Date: Day:

	Wake	Breakfast	Lunch	Dinner	Bed
Before					
After					
Notes:					

Date: Day:

	Wake	Breakfast	Lunch	Dinner	Bed
Before					
After					
Notes:					

Date: Day:

	Wake	Breakfast	Lunch	Dinner	Bed
Before					
After					
Notes:					

Date: Day:

	Wake	Breakfast	Lunch	Dinner	Bed
Before					
After					
Notes:					

Date: Day:

	Wake	Breakfast	Lunch	Dinner	Bed
Before					
After					
Notes:					

Date: Day:

	Wake	Breakfast	Lunch	Dinner	Bed
Before					
After					
Notes:					

Date: Day:

	Wake	Breakfast	Lunch	Dinner	Bed
Before					
After					
Notes:					

Date: Day:

	Wake	Breakfast	Lunch	Dinner	Bed
Before					
After					
Notes:					

Date: Day:

	Wake	Breakfast	Lunch	Dinner	Bed
Before					
After					
Notes:					

Date: Day:

	Wake	Breakfast	Lunch	Dinner	Bed
Before					
After					
Notes:					

Date: Day:

	Wake	Breakfast	Lunch	Dinner	Bed
Before					
After					
Notes:					

Date: Day:

	Wake	Breakfast	Lunch	Dinner	Bed
Before					
After					
Notes:					

Date: Day:

	Wake	Breakfast	Lunch	Dinner	Bed
Before					
After					
Notes:					

Date: Day:

	Wake	Breakfast	Lunch	Dinner	Bed
Before					
After					
Notes:					

Date: Day:

	Wake	Breakfast	Lunch	Dinner	Bed
Before					
After					
Notes:					

Date: Day:

	Wake	Breakfast	Lunch	Dinner	Bed
Before					
After					
Notes:					

Date: Day:

	Wake	Breakfast	Lunch	Dinner	Bed
Before					
After					
Notes:					

Date: Day:

	Wake	Breakfast	Lunch	Dinner	Bed
Before					
After					
Notes:					

Date: Day:

	Wake	Breakfast	Lunch	Dinner	Bed
Before					
After					
Notes:					

Date: Day:

	Wake	Breakfast	Lunch	Dinner	Bed
Before					
After					
Notes:					

Date: Day:

	Wake	Breakfast	Lunch	Dinner	Bed
Before					
After					
Notes:					

Date: Day:

	Wake	Breakfast	Lunch	Dinner	Bed
Before					
After					
Notes:					

Date: Day:

	Wake	Breakfast	Lunch	Dinner	Bed
Before					
After					
Notes:					

Date: Day:

	Wake	Breakfast	Lunch	Dinner	Bed
Before					
After					
Notes:					

Date: Day:

	Wake	Breakfast	Lunch	Dinner	Bed
Before					
After					
Notes:					

Date: Day:

	Wake	Breakfast	Lunch	Dinner	Bed
Before					
After					
Notes:					

Date: Day:

	Wake	Breakfast	Lunch	Dinner	Bed
Before					
After					
Notes:					

Date: Day:

	Wake	Breakfast	Lunch	Dinner	Bed
Before					
After					
Notes:					

Date: Day:

	Wake	Breakfast	Lunch	Dinner	Bed
Before					
After					
Notes:					

Date: Day:

	Wake	Breakfast	Lunch	Dinner	Bed
Before					
After					
Notes:					

Date: Day:

	Wake	Breakfast	Lunch	Dinner	Bed
Before					
After					
Notes:					

Date: Day:

	Wake	Breakfast	Lunch	Dinner	Bed
Before					
After					
Notes:					

Date: Day:

	Wake	Breakfast	Lunch	Dinner	Bed
Before					
After					
Notes:					

Date: Day:

	Wake	Breakfast	Lunch	Dinner	Bed
Before					
After					
Notes:					

Date: Day:

	Wake	Breakfast	Lunch	Dinner	Bed
Before					
After					
Notes:					

Date: Day:

	Wake	Breakfast	Lunch	Dinner	Bed
Before					
After					
Notes:					

Date: Day:

	Wake	Breakfast	Lunch	Dinner	Bed
Before					
After					
Notes:					

Date: Day:

	Wake	Breakfast	Lunch	Dinner	Bed
Before					
After					
Notes:					

Date: Day:

	Wake	Breakfast	Lunch	Dinner	Bed
Before					
After					
Notes:					

Date: Day:

	Wake	Breakfast	Lunch	Dinner	Bed
Before					
After					
Notes:					

Date: Day:

	Wake	Breakfast	Lunch	Dinner	Bed
Before					
After					
Notes:					

Date: Day:

	Wake	Breakfast	Lunch	Dinner	Bed
Before					
After					
Notes:					

Date: Day:

	Wake	Breakfast	Lunch	Dinner	Bed
Before					
After					
Notes:					

Date: Day:

	Wake	Breakfast	Lunch	Dinner	Bed
Before					
After					
Notes:					

Date: Day:

	Wake	Breakfast	Lunch	Dinner	Bed
Before					
After					
Notes:					

Date: Day:

	Wake	Breakfast	Lunch	Dinner	Bed
Before					
After					
Notes:					

Date: Day:

	Wake	Breakfast	Lunch	Dinner	Bed
Before					
After					
Notes:					

Date: Day:

	Wake	Breakfast	Lunch	Dinner	Bed
Before					
After					
Notes:					

Date: Day:

	Wake	Breakfast	Lunch	Dinner	Bed
Before					
After					
Notes:					

Date: Day:

	Wake	Breakfast	Lunch	Dinner	Bed
Before					
After					
Notes:					

Date: Day:

	Wake	Breakfast	Lunch	Dinner	Bed
Before					
After					
Notes:					

Date: Day:

	Wake	Breakfast	Lunch	Dinner	Bed
Before					
After					
Notes:					

Date: Day:

	Wake	Breakfast	Lunch	Dinner	Bed
Before					
After					
Notes:					

Date: Day:

	Wake	Breakfast	Lunch	Dinner	Bed
Before					
After					
Notes:					

Date: Day:

	Wake	Breakfast	Lunch	Dinner	Bed
Before					
After					
Notes:					

Date: Day:

	Wake	Breakfast	Lunch	Dinner	Bed
Before					
After					
Notes:					

Date: Day:

	Wake	Breakfast	Lunch	Dinner	Bed
Before					
After					
Notes:					

Date: Day:

	Wake	Breakfast	Lunch	Dinner	Bed
Before					
After					
Notes:					

Date: Day:

	Wake	Breakfast	Lunch	Dinner	Bed
Before					
After					
Notes:					

Date: Day:

	Wake	Breakfast	Lunch	Dinner	Bed
Before					
After					
Notes:					

Date: Day:

	Wake	Breakfast	Lunch	Dinner	Bed
Before					
After					
Notes:					

Date: Day:

	Wake	Breakfast	Lunch	Dinner	Bed
Before					
After					
Notes:					

Date: Day:

	Wake	Breakfast	Lunch	Dinner	Bed
Before					
After					
Notes:					

Date: Day:

	Wake	Breakfast	Lunch	Dinner	Bed
Before					
After					
Notes:					

Date: Day:

	Wake	Breakfast	Lunch	Dinner	Bed
Before					
After					
Notes:					

Date: Day:

	Wake	Breakfast	Lunch	Dinner	Bed
Before					
After					
Notes:					

Date: Day:

	Wake	Breakfast	Lunch	Dinner	Bed
Before					
After					
Notes:					

Date: Day:

	Wake	Breakfast	Lunch	Dinner	Bed
Before					
After					
Notes:					

Date: Day:

	Wake	Breakfast	Lunch	Dinner	Bed
Before					
After					
Notes:					

Date: Day:

	Wake	Breakfast	Lunch	Dinner	Bed
Before					
After					
Notes:					

Date: Day:

	Wake	Breakfast	Lunch	Dinner	Bed
Before					
After					
Notes:					

Date: Day:

	Wake	Breakfast	Lunch	Dinner	Bed
Before					
After					
Notes:					

Date: Day:

	Wake	Breakfast	Lunch	Dinner	Bed
Before					
After					
Notes:					

Date: Day:

	Wake	Breakfast	Lunch	Dinner	Bed
Before					
After					
Notes:					

Date: Day:

	Wake	Breakfast	Lunch	Dinner	Bed
Before					
After					
Notes:					

Date: Day:

	Wake	Breakfast	Lunch	Dinner	Bed
Before					
After					
Notes:					

Date: Day:

	Wake	Breakfast	Lunch	Dinner	Bed
Before					
After					
Notes:					

Date: Day:

	Wake	Breakfast	Lunch	Dinner	Bed
Before					
After					
Notes:					

Date: Day:

	Wake	Breakfast	Lunch	Dinner	Bed
Before					
After					
Notes:					

Date: Day:

	Wake	Breakfast	Lunch	Dinner	Bed
Before					
After					
Notes:					

Date: Day:

	Wake	Breakfast	Lunch	Dinner	Bed
Before					
After					
Notes:					

Date: Day:

	Wake	Breakfast	Lunch	Dinner	Bed
Before					
After					
Notes:					

Date: Day:

	Wake	Breakfast	Lunch	Dinner	Bed
Before					
After					
Notes:					

Date: Day:

	Wake	Breakfast	Lunch	Dinner	Bed
Before					
After					
Notes:					

Date: Day:

	Wake	Breakfast	Lunch	Dinner	Bed
Before					
After					
Notes:					

Date: Day:

	Wake	Breakfast	Lunch	Dinner	Bed
Before					
After					
Notes:					

Date: Day:

	Wake	Breakfast	Lunch	Dinner	Bed
Before					
After					
Notes:					

Date: Day:

	Wake	Breakfast	Lunch	Dinner	Bed
Before					
After					
Notes:					

Date: Day:

	Wake	Breakfast	Lunch	Dinner	Bed
Before					
After					
Notes:					

Date: Day:

	Wake	Breakfast	Lunch	Dinner	Bed
Before					
After					
Notes:					

Date: Day:

	Wake	Breakfast	Lunch	Dinner	Bed
Before					
After					
Notes:					

Date: Day:

	Wake	Breakfast	Lunch	Dinner	Bed
Before					
After					
Notes:					

Date: Day:

	Wake	Breakfast	Lunch	Dinner	Bed
Before					
After					
Notes:					

Date: Day:

	Wake	Breakfast	Lunch	Dinner	Bed
Before					
After					
Notes:					

Date: Day:

	Wake	Breakfast	Lunch	Dinner	Bed
Before					
After					
Notes:					

Date: Day:

	Wake	Breakfast	Lunch	Dinner	Bed
Before					
After					
Notes:					

Date: Day:

	Wake	Breakfast	Lunch	Dinner	Bed
Before					
After					
Notes:					

Date: Day:

	Wake	Breakfast	Lunch	Dinner	Bed
Before					
After					
Notes:					

Date: Day:

	Wake	Breakfast	Lunch	Dinner	Bed
Before					
After					
Notes:					

Date: Day:

	Wake	Breakfast	Lunch	Dinner	Bed
Before					
After					
Notes:					

Date: Day:

	Wake	Breakfast	Lunch	Dinner	Bed
Before					
After					
Notes:					

Date: Day:

	Wake	Breakfast	Lunch	Dinner	Bed
Before					
After					
Notes:					

Date: Day:

	Wake	Breakfast	Lunch	Dinner	Bed
Before					
After					
Notes:					

Date: Day:

	Wake	Breakfast	Lunch	Dinner	Bed
Before					
After					
Notes:					

Date: Day:

	Wake	Breakfast	Lunch	Dinner	Bed
Before					
After					
Notes:					

Date: Day:

	Wake	Breakfast	Lunch	Dinner	Bed
Before					
After					
Notes:					

Date: Day:

	Wake	Breakfast	Lunch	Dinner	Bed
Before					
After					
Notes:					

Date: Day:

	Wake	Breakfast	Lunch	Dinner	Bed
Before					
After					
Notes:					

Date: Day:

	Wake	Breakfast	Lunch	Dinner	Bed
Before					
After					
Notes:					

Date: Day:

	Wake	Breakfast	Lunch	Dinner	Bed
Before					
After					
Notes:					

Date: Day:

	Wake	Breakfast	Lunch	Dinner	Bed
Before					
After					
Notes:					

Date: Day:

	Wake	Breakfast	Lunch	Dinner	Bed
Before					
After					
Notes:					

Date: Day:

	Wake	Breakfast	Lunch	Dinner	Bed
Before					
After					
Notes:					

Date: Day:

	Wake	Breakfast	Lunch	Dinner	Bed
Before					
After					
Notes:					

Date: Day:

	Wake	Breakfast	Lunch	Dinner	Bed
Before					
After					
Notes:					

Date: Day:

	Wake	Breakfast	Lunch	Dinner	Bed
Before					
After					
Notes:					

Date: Day:

	Wake	Breakfast	Lunch	Dinner	Bed
Before					
After					
Notes:					

Date: Day:

	Wake	Breakfast	Lunch	Dinner	Bed
Before					
After					
Notes:					

Date: Day:

	Wake	Breakfast	Lunch	Dinner	Bed
Before					
After					
Notes:					

Date: Day:

	Wake	Breakfast	Lunch	Dinner	Bed
Before					
After					
Notes:					

Date: Day:

	Wake	Breakfast	Lunch	Dinner	Bed
Before					
After					
Notes:					

Date: Day:

	Wake	Breakfast	Lunch	Dinner	Bed
Before					
After					
Notes:					

Date: Day:

	Wake	Breakfast	Lunch	Dinner	Bed
Before					
After					
Notes:					

Date: Day:

	Wake	Breakfast	Lunch	Dinner	Bed
Before					
After					
Notes:					

Date: Day:

	Wake	Breakfast	Lunch	Dinner	Bed
Before					
After					
Notes:					

Date: Day:

	Wake	Breakfast	Lunch	Dinner	Bed
Before					
After					
Notes:					

Date: Day:

	Wake	Breakfast	Lunch	Dinner	Bed
Before					
After					
Notes:					

Date: Day:

	Wake	Breakfast	Lunch	Dinner	Bed
Before					
After					
Notes:					

Date: Day:

	Wake	Breakfast	Lunch	Dinner	Bed
Before					
After					
Notes:					

Date: Day:

	Wake	Breakfast	Lunch	Dinner	Bed
Before					
After					
Notes:					

Date: Day:

	Wake	Breakfast	Lunch	Dinner	Bed
Before					
After					
Notes:					

Date: Day:

	Wake	Breakfast	Lunch	Dinner	Bed
Before					
After					
Notes:					

Date: Day:

	Wake	Breakfast	Lunch	Dinner	Bed
Before					
After					
Notes:					

Date: Day:

	Wake	Breakfast	Lunch	Dinner	Bed
Before					
After					
Notes:					

Date: Day:

	Wake	Breakfast	Lunch	Dinner	Bed
Before					
After					
Notes:					

Date: Day:

	Wake	Breakfast	Lunch	Dinner	Bed
Before					
After					
Notes:					

Date: Day:

	Wake	Breakfast	Lunch	Dinner	Bed
Before					
After					
Notes:					

Date: Day:

	Wake	Breakfast	Lunch	Dinner	Bed
Before					
After					
Notes:					

Date: Day:

	Wake	Breakfast	Lunch	Dinner	Bed
Before					
After					
Notes:					

Date: Day:

	Wake	Breakfast	Lunch	Dinner	Bed
Before					
After					
Notes:					

Date: Day:

	Wake	Breakfast	Lunch	Dinner	Bed
Before					
After					
Notes:					

Date: Day:

	Wake	Breakfast	Lunch	Dinner	Bed
Before					
After					
Notes:					

Date: Day:

	Wake	Breakfast	Lunch	Dinner	Bed
Before					
After					
Notes:					

Date: Day:

	Wake	Breakfast	Lunch	Dinner	Bed
Before					
After					
Notes:					

Date: Day:

	Wake	Breakfast	Lunch	Dinner	Bed
Before					
After					
Notes:					

Date: Day:

	Wake	Breakfast	Lunch	Dinner	Bed
Before					
After					
Notes:					

Date: Day:

	Wake	Breakfast	Lunch	Dinner	Bed
Before					
After					
Notes:					

Date: Day:

	Wake	Breakfast	Lunch	Dinner	Bed
Before					
After					
Notes:					

Date: Day:

	Wake	Breakfast	Lunch	Dinner	Bed
Before					
After					
Notes:					

Date: Day:

	Wake	Breakfast	Lunch	Dinner	Bed
Before					
After					
Notes:					

Date: Day:

	Wake	Breakfast	Lunch	Dinner	Bed
Before					
After					
Notes:					

Date: Day:

	Wake	Breakfast	Lunch	Dinner	Bed
Before					
After					
Notes:					

Date: Day:

	Wake	Breakfast	Lunch	Dinner	Bed
Before					
After					
Notes:					

Date: Day:

	Wake	Breakfast	Lunch	Dinner	Bed
Before					
After					
Notes:					

Date: Day:

	Wake	Breakfast	Lunch	Dinner	Bed
Before					
After					
Notes:					

Date: Day:

	Wake	Breakfast	Lunch	Dinner	Bed
Before					
After					
Notes:					

Date: Day:

	Wake	Breakfast	Lunch	Dinner	Bed
Before					
After					
Notes:					

Date: Day:

	Wake	Breakfast	Lunch	Dinner	Bed
Before					
After					
Notes:					

Date: Day:

	Wake	Breakfast	Lunch	Dinner	Bed
Before					
After					
Notes:					

Date: Day:

	Wake	Breakfast	Lunch	Dinner	Bed
Before					
After					
Notes:					

Date: Day:

	Wake	Breakfast	Lunch	Dinner	Bed
Before					
After					
Notes:					

Date: Day:

	Wake	Breakfast	Lunch	Dinner	Bed
Before					
After					
Notes:					

Date: Day:

	Wake	Breakfast	Lunch	Dinner	Bed
Before					
After					
Notes:					

Date: Day:

	Wake	Breakfast	Lunch	Dinner	Bed
Before					
After					
Notes:					

Date: Day:

	Wake	Breakfast	Lunch	Dinner	Bed
Before					
After					
Notes:					

Date: Day:

	Wake	Breakfast	Lunch	Dinner	Bed
Before					
After					
Notes:					

Date: Day:

	Wake	Breakfast	Lunch	Dinner	Bed
Before					
After					
Notes:					

Date: Day:

	Wake	Breakfast	Lunch	Dinner	Bed
Before					
After					
Notes:					

Date: Day:

	Wake	Breakfast	Lunch	Dinner	Bed
Before					
After					
Notes:					

Date: Day:

	Wake	Breakfast	Lunch	Dinner	Bed
Before					
After					
Notes:					

Date: Day:

	Wake	Breakfast	Lunch	Dinner	Bed
Before					
After					
Notes:					

Date: Day:

	Wake	Breakfast	Lunch	Dinner	Bed
Before					
After					
Notes:					

Date: Day:

	Wake	Breakfast	Lunch	Dinner	Bed
Before					
After					
Notes:					

Date: Day:

	Wake	Breakfast	Lunch	Dinner	Bed
Before					
After					
Notes:					

Date: Day:

	Wake	Breakfast	Lunch	Dinner	Bed
Before					
After					
Notes:					

Date: Day:

	Wake	Breakfast	Lunch	Dinner	Bed
Before					
After					
Notes:					

Date: Day:

	Wake	Breakfast	Lunch	Dinner	Bed
Before					
After					
Notes:					

Date: Day:

	Wake	Breakfast	Lunch	Dinner	Bed
Before					
After					
Notes:					

Date: Day:

	Wake	Breakfast	Lunch	Dinner	Bed
Before					
After					
Notes:					

Date: Day:

	Wake	Breakfast	Lunch	Dinner	Bed
Before					
After					
Notes:					

Date: Day:

	Wake	Breakfast	Lunch	Dinner	Bed
Before					
After					
Notes:					

Date: Day:

	Wake	Breakfast	Lunch	Dinner	Bed
Before					
After					
Notes:					

Date: Day:

	Wake	Breakfast	Lunch	Dinner	Bed
Before					
After					
Notes:					

Date: Day:

	Wake	Breakfast	Lunch	Dinner	Bed
Before					
After					
Notes:					

Date: Day:

	Wake	Breakfast	Lunch	Dinner	Bed
Before					
After					
Notes:					

Date: Day:

	Wake	Breakfast	Lunch	Dinner	Bed
Before					
After					
Notes:					

Date: Day:

	Wake	Breakfast	Lunch	Dinner	Bed
Before					
After					
Notes:					

Date: Day:

	Wake	Breakfast	Lunch	Dinner	Bed
Before					
After					
Notes:					

Date: Day:

	Wake	Breakfast	Lunch	Dinner	Bed
Before					
After					
Notes:					

Date: Day:

	Wake	Breakfast	Lunch	Dinner	Bed
Before					
After					
Notes:					

Date: Day:

	Wake	Breakfast	Lunch	Dinner	Bed
Before					
After					
Notes:					

Date: Day:

	Wake	Breakfast	Lunch	Dinner	Bed
Before					
After					
Notes:					

Date: Day:

	Wake	Breakfast	Lunch	Dinner	Bed
Before					
After					
Notes:					

Date: Day:

	Wake	Breakfast	Lunch	Dinner	Bed
Before					
After					
Notes:					

Date: Day:

	Wake	Breakfast	Lunch	Dinner	Bed
Before					
After					
Notes:					

Date: Day:

	Wake	Breakfast	Lunch	Dinner	Bed
Before					
After					
Notes:					

Date: Day:

	Wake	Breakfast	Lunch	Dinner	Bed
Before					
After					
Notes:					

Date: Day:

	Wake	Breakfast	Lunch	Dinner	Bed
Before					
After					
Notes:					

Date: Day:

	Wake	Breakfast	Lunch	Dinner	Bed
Before					
After					
Notes:					

Date: Day:

	Wake	Breakfast	Lunch	Dinner	Bed
Before					
After					
Notes:					

Date: Day:

	Wake	Breakfast	Lunch	Dinner	Bed
Before					
After					
Notes:					

Date: Day:

	Wake	Breakfast	Lunch	Dinner	Bed
Before					
After					
Notes:					

Date: Day:

	Wake	Breakfast	Lunch	Dinner	Bed
Before					
After					
Notes:					

Date: Day:

	Wake	Breakfast	Lunch	Dinner	Bed
Before					
After					
Notes:					

Date: Day:

	Wake	Breakfast	Lunch	Dinner	Bed
Before					
After					
Notes:					

Date: Day:

	Wake	Breakfast	Lunch	Dinner	Bed
Before					
After					
Notes:					

Date: Day:

	Wake	Breakfast	Lunch	Dinner	Bed
Before					
After					
Notes:					

Date: Day:

	Wake	Breakfast	Lunch	Dinner	Bed
Before					
After					
Notes:					

Date: Day:

	Wake	Breakfast	Lunch	Dinner	Bed
Before					
After					
Notes:					

Date: Day:

	Wake	Breakfast	Lunch	Dinner	Bed
Before					
After					
Notes:					

Date: Day:

	Wake	Breakfast	Lunch	Dinner	Bed
Before					
After					
Notes:					

Date: Day:

	Wake	Breakfast	Lunch	Dinner	Bed
Before					
After					
Notes:					

Date: Day:

	Wake	Breakfast	Lunch	Dinner	Bed
Before					
After					
Notes:					

Date: Day:

	Wake	Breakfast	Lunch	Dinner	Bed
Before					
After					
Notes:					

Date: Day:

	Wake	Breakfast	Lunch	Dinner	Bed
Before					
After					
Notes:					

Date: Day:

	Wake	Breakfast	Lunch	Dinner	Bed
Before					
After					
Notes:					

Date: Day:

	Wake	Breakfast	Lunch	Dinner	Bed
Before					
After					
Notes:					

Date: Day:

	Wake	Breakfast	Lunch	Dinner	Bed
Before					
After					
Notes:					

Date: Day:

	Wake	Breakfast	Lunch	Dinner	Bed
Before					
After					
Notes:					

Date: Day:

	Wake	Breakfast	Lunch	Dinner	Bed
Before					
After					
Notes:					

Date: Day:

	Wake	Breakfast	Lunch	Dinner	Bed
Before					
After					
Notes:					

Date: Day:

	Wake	Breakfast	Lunch	Dinner	Bed
Before					
After					
Notes:					

Date: Day:

	Wake	Breakfast	Lunch	Dinner	Bed
Before					
After					
Notes:					

Date: Day:

	Wake	Breakfast	Lunch	Dinner	Bed
Before					
After					
Notes:					

Date: Day:

	Wake	Breakfast	Lunch	Dinner	Bed
Before					
After					
Notes:					

Date: Day:

	Wake	Breakfast	Lunch	Dinner	Bed
Before					
After					
Notes:					

Date: Day:

	Wake	Breakfast	Lunch	Dinner	Bed
Before					
After					
Notes:					

Date: Day:

	Wake	Breakfast	Lunch	Dinner	Bed
Before					
After					
Notes:					

Date: Day:

	Wake	Breakfast	Lunch	Dinner	Bed
Before					
After					
Notes:					

Date: Day:

	Wake	Breakfast	Lunch	Dinner	Bed
Before					
After					
Notes:					

Date: Day:

	Wake	Breakfast	Lunch	Dinner	Bed
Before					
After					
Notes:					

Date: Day:

	Wake	Breakfast	Lunch	Dinner	Bed
Before					
After					
Notes:					

Date: Day:

	Wake	Breakfast	Lunch	Dinner	Bed
Before					
After					
Notes:					

Date: Day:

	Wake	Breakfast	Lunch	Dinner	Bed
Before					
After					
Notes:					

Date: Day:

	Wake	Breakfast	Lunch	Dinner	Bed
Before					
After					
Notes:					

Date: Day:

	Wake	Breakfast	Lunch	Dinner	Bed
Before					
After					
Notes:					

Date: Day:

	Wake	Breakfast	Lunch	Dinner	Bed
Before					
After					
Notes:					

Date: Day:

	Wake	Breakfast	Lunch	Dinner	Bed
Before					
After					
Notes:					

Date: Day:

	Wake	Breakfast	Lunch	Dinner	Bed
Before					
After					
Notes:					

Date: Day:

	Wake	Breakfast	Lunch	Dinner	Bed
Before					
After					
Notes:					

Date: Day:

	Wake	Breakfast	Lunch	Dinner	Bed
Before					
After					
Notes:					

Date: Day:

	Wake	Breakfast	Lunch	Dinner	Bed
Before					
After					
Notes:					

Date: Day:

	Wake	Breakfast	Lunch	Dinner	Bed
Before					
After					
Notes:					

Date: Day:

	Wake	Breakfast	Lunch	Dinner	Bed
Before					
After					
Notes:					

Date: Day:

	Wake	Breakfast	Lunch	Dinner	Bed
Before					
After					
Notes:					

Date: Day:

	Wake	Breakfast	Lunch	Dinner	Bed
Before					
After					
Notes:					

Date: Day:

	Wake	Breakfast	Lunch	Dinner	Bed
Before					
After					
Notes:					

Date: Day:

	Wake	Breakfast	Lunch	Dinner	Bed
Before					
After					
Notes:					

Date: Day:

	Wake	Breakfast	Lunch	Dinner	Bed
Before					
After					
Notes:					

Date: Day:

	Wake	Breakfast	Lunch	Dinner	Bed
Before					
After					
Notes:					

Date: Day:

	Wake	Breakfast	Lunch	Dinner	Bed
Before					
After					
Notes:					

Date: Day:

	Wake	Breakfast	Lunch	Dinner	Bed
Before					
After					
Notes:					

Date: Day:

	Wake	Breakfast	Lunch	Dinner	Bed
Before					
After					
Notes:					

Date: Day:

	Wake	Breakfast	Lunch	Dinner	Bed
Before					
After					
Notes:					

Date: Day:

	Wake	Breakfast	Lunch	Dinner	Bed
Before					
After					
Notes:					

Date: Day:

	Wake	Breakfast	Lunch	Dinner	Bed
Before					
After					
Notes:					

Date: Day:

	Wake	Breakfast	Lunch	Dinner	Bed
Before					
After					
Notes:					

Date: Day:

	Wake	Breakfast	Lunch	Dinner	Bed
Before					
After					
Notes:					

Date: Day:

	Wake	Breakfast	Lunch	Dinner	Bed
Before					
After					
Notes:					

Date: Day:

	Wake	Breakfast	Lunch	Dinner	Bed
Before					
After					
Notes:					

Date: Day:

	Wake	Breakfast	Lunch	Dinner	Bed
Before					
After					
Notes:					

Date: Day:

	Wake	Breakfast	Lunch	Dinner	Bed
Before					
After					
Notes:					

Date: Day:

	Wake	Breakfast	Lunch	Dinner	Bed
Before					
After					
Notes:					

Date: Day:

	Wake	Breakfast	Lunch	Dinner	Bed
Before					
After					
Notes:					

Date: Day:

	Wake	Breakfast	Lunch	Dinner	Bed
Before					
After					
Notes:					

Date: Day:

	Wake	Breakfast	Lunch	Dinner	Bed
Before					
After					
Notes:					

Date: Day:

	Wake	Breakfast	Lunch	Dinner	Bed
Before					
After					
Notes:					

Date: Day:

	Wake	Breakfast	Lunch	Dinner	Bed
Before					
After					
Notes:					

Date: Day:

	Wake	Breakfast	Lunch	Dinner	Bed
Before					
After					
Notes:					

Date: Day:

	Wake	Breakfast	Lunch	Dinner	Bed
Before					
After					
Notes:					

Date: Day:

	Wake	Breakfast	Lunch	Dinner	Bed
Before					
After					
Notes:					

Date: Day:

	Wake	Breakfast	Lunch	Dinner	Bed
Before					
After					
Notes:					

Date: Day:

	Wake	Breakfast	Lunch	Dinner	Bed
Before					
After					
Notes:					

Date: Day:

	Wake	Breakfast	Lunch	Dinner	Bed
Before					
After					
Notes:					

Date: Day:

	Wake	Breakfast	Lunch	Dinner	Bed
Before					
After					
Notes:					

Date: Day:

	Wake	Breakfast	Lunch	Dinner	Bed
Before					
After					
Notes:					

Date: Day:

	Wake	Breakfast	Lunch	Dinner	Bed
Before					
After					
Notes:					

Date: Day:

	Wake	Breakfast	Lunch	Dinner	Bed
Before					
After					
Notes:					

www.ingramcontent.com/pod-product-compliance
Lightning Source LLC
Chambersburg PA
CBHW070424290526
45791CB00005B/1824